The Virgin Extensions

Hair Care Manual

A Step By Step Guide To Maintaining Healthy Hair Extensions

AUTHOR BREANNA RUTTER

TABLE OF CONTENTS

THE VIRGIN EXTENSIONS HAIR CARE MANUAL

INTRODUCTION TO THE VIRGIN EXTENSIONS HAIR CARE MANUAL

"The Virgin Extensions Hair Care Manual is a step by step guide that will help you to take care & maintain healthy hair extensions. Depending on the quality of your hair extensions, taking care of them can take little or demanding effort to maintain its integrity. With the knowledge you may already have, you probably have already experienced dry hair, split ends, or even heat damaged hair ruining yet another set of hair extensions! This makes caring for your extensions very challenging & frustrating considering the price you pay for your investment of hair!

In this manual, I promise to provide step by step instructions on caring for your virgin hair extensions. Even if you do not have virgin hair extensions, all of the information shared in this manual is still applicable but keep in mind that the quality of your hair extensions directly influences its life span despite your healthy hair care practices!

In this manual, I promise to guide you to your best hair care products & styling tools to be used on your hair extensions for your styling & maintenance needs. Additionally, I will also give you step by step instructions on how to use your hairstyling tools & hair care products to give you beautiful results with your hair!

Enjoy this informative read, I know you will love this!"

Sincerely, Breanna

1 HAIR CARE TOOLS

It should be of no surprise that the tools you use to detangle & groom your hair are extremely important in regards to maintaining the health of your hair extensions. We can easily become consumed by finding the perfect hair care products for our extensions, even for our real hair, while forgetting to pay attention to the unforgettable damage caused by inappropriate hair care tools! The only hair tool that is necessary in maintaining healthy hair extensions is a wide tooth comb/detangling comb! This has always been the #1 secret to great hair no matter how fine, thick, course, silky, curly, straight, or wavy your hair extensions are, you will always need a wide tooth comb for your detangling & grooming needs! This is how you will forever prevent a great deal of damage & split ends, trust me!

What's also just as important as a seamless detangling comb are a pair of hair cutting shears! The beauty about quality hair extensions is that the hair is already in tip top condition since it is virgin hair & the flip side to this is that since it is real high quality hair, it's natural to experience damaged or splitting ends. Damaged or splitting ends happen to every one of us but maintenance prevents this from spiraling out of control! Real hair overtime, naturally becomes drier & courser near the ends (since this is the oldest part of your hair) so it's a given that you will experience split ends or slightly damaged ends even if you have very healthy hair! The very same thing applies to extensions so trimming the ends occasionally is necessary for maintaining healthy hair extensions.

I will walk you step by step through how to trim the ends of your extensions to keep them healthy & free from damage!

Trimming Regimen For Removable Extensions

Step #1 Begin with clean dry extensions that has been shampooed & deep conditioned.

Do not add any hair products to your extensions! Product weighs down your ends which causes some splitting/damaged hairs to be missed after trimming. Hair products slick down your hair & once the product is removed, you will notice your split ends again!

Step #2 Gather a section that has the same length of hair & ponytail it. You should have ponytails all over your head! Working on one ponytail at a time, comb your extensions straight down with a wide tooth comb. This prevents a choppy look especially with layered extensions!

Step #3 Take a thin small amount of hair from the ponytail you are working on & use a clip to keep the rest of the loose hair separate. Loosely grip the small section of hair between your index & middle finger of your less dominant hand & trim horizontally about 1/8 inch of hair with your dominant hand.

After trimming any section, use a hair clip to keep trimmed hair separate from hair that has not been trimmed yet.

Trimming the hair over a waste basket catches the hair clippings & allows gravity to naturally elongate your extensions to help you trim the intended amount of hair.

Trimming Regimen For Non Removable Extensions

Step #1 Begin with clean dry extensions that has been shampooed & deep conditioned.

Do not add any hair products to your extensions! Product weighs down your ends which causes some splitting/ damaged hairs to be missed after trimming. Hair products slick down your hair & once the product is removed, you will notice your split ends again!

Step #2 Gather a section that has the same length of hair & ponytail it. You should have ponytails all over your head! Working on one ponytail at a time, comb your extensions straight down with a wide tooth comb. This prevents a choppy look especially with layered extensions! Keep your real hair sectioned away!

Step #3 Take a thin small amount of hair from the ponytail you are working on & use a clip to keep the rest of the loose hair separate. Loosely grip the small section of hair between your index & middle finger of your less dominant hand & trim horizontally about 1/8 inch of hair with your dominant hand.

After trimming any section, use a hair clip to keep trimmed hair separate from hair that has not been trimmed yet.

Trimming the hair over a waste basket catches the hair clippings & allows gravity to naturally elongate your extensions to help you trim the intended amount of hair.

SAFE HAIR CARE TOOLS	HARSH HAIR CARE TOOLS
Seamless Wide Tooth Combs	Combs with Seams
Soft Boar Bristle Hair Brush	Plastic Bristle Hair Brush
Hair Cutting Shears (only to be used on extensions)	Safety Scissors (Household Scissors)

2 DETANGLE

Keeping your hair extensions groomed stops your extensions from becoming tangled or even worse & sometimes irreversible, matted! It's extremely easy to keep your extensions free of tangles & to do so, you simply want to detangle the hair, at least daily, with a wide tooth comb! Sometimes just simply raking your fingers gently through your hair is enough! If you find yourself excessively detangling your hair extensions throughout the day, you have to know the quality of your extensions to avoid these problems. Sad to say but expensive hair extensions can still be of poor quality. Hair extensions that tangle very easily & commonly mat where there is friction (like the area behind your neck) is an obvious indication that you do not have quality hair extensions.

Detangling your hair extensions will differ depending on how tight of a curl your extensions are. Straight to wavy hair should be detangled while dry instead of wet. Curly to coily hair should be detangled wet instead of dry. To keep your curls/coils looking fresh & frizz-free throughout the day, you should not detangle your hair or rake your fingers through your curls especially when dry! Only detangle curly to coily hair while wet or damp with conditioner. Also as tempting as it may be, refrain from handling curly to coily hair while drying & dry to preserve neat looking extensions.

I will walk you step by step through how to detangle your hair properly no matter the texture or curl pattern of your virgin hair extensions!

Detangling Regimen For Straight to Wavy Hair
(Removable & Non Removable Extensions)

Detangle extensions in manageable sections from the tips to the roots with a seamless wide tooth comb/detangling comb. If applicable, you can opt to finger detangle instead.

Detangling Regimen For Curly to Coily Hair
(Removable & Non Removable Extensions)

Step#1 Generously apply water & conditioner to your extensions. If applicable secure away your real hair.

Step #2 Detangle extensions in manageable sections from the tips to the roots with a seamless wide tooth detangling comb.

Step #3 Allow warm water to wash the conditioner out of the hair. Refrain from manipulating or handling your curls/coils while & after rinsing out the conditioner.

Final rinse with the coolest water you can stand for smooth shiny hair.

Step #4 (Non Removable Extensions)
Gently scrunch towel dry curls/coils & allow to air dry with an absorbent towel around your neck.

(Removable Extensions) Hang dry your extensions on pant hangers or dry on top of an absorbent towel.

3 SHAMPOO

For some, shampoo washing your hair extensions can be the ultimate test to determine the true quality of your hair! Nonetheless, shampoo washing your extensions is necessary when maintaining healthy virgin hair extensions. Applying shampoo to your extensions should never cause them to become tangled or matted if they are of quality! Before shampoo washing your hair, it is very important that the hair has been detangled prior no matter the texture & curl pattern for best results. Shampooing extensions that have not been detangled will only cause more tangles. Straight to wavy hair is a little bit more forgiving to be shampooed without detangling than curly to coily hair but taking that chance can be extremely detrimental to your hair extensions! No matter what, you have to detangle your hair before shampooing always!

A good guide for knowing how often to shampoo wash your hair extensions is at least once or twice a week. This will vary depending on the frequency of your hair product usage & the quality of your hair extensions. You can choose to shampoo wash your extensions by paying attention to notice a buildup of hair products, dead skin flakes or even an odor. Shampoo your extensions only to cleanse the hair of such buildups. Conditioner washing or moisturizing is the more applicable option if you are only in need of moisture instead of cleansing. After shampooing your hair you have to follow up with a moisturizer.

I will walk you step by step through how to shampoo wash your hair extensions properly from start to finish!

If you are in need of a quality shampoo for your extensions, I highly suggest referring to HowToBlackHair.com for suggested product needs.

Shampoo Regimen
(Removable & Non Removable Extensions)

Step#1 Implement the detangle regimen according to what is applicable for your type of hair extensions.

If applicable, separate & secure away your real hair from your extensions.

Step #2 Lather shampoo in your hands & then apply the lather to your extensions.

Thoroughly message hair & binding of your hair extensions with the shampoo lather.

Step #3 Allow warm water to wash the shampoo out of your hair extensions.

Refrain from manipulating or handling your hair while & after rinsing out the shampoo.

Final rinse with the coolest water you can stand for smooth shiny hair.

Step #4 (Non Removable Extensions)
Gently scrunch towel dry extensions & allow to air dry with an absorbent towel around your neck.

(Removable Extensions) Hang dry your extensions on pant hangers or dry on top of an absorbent towel.

4 DEEP CONDITION

Overtime, your extensions will naturally wear & tear so deep condition treatments are necessary from time to time. Through styling practices & daily manipulation, the hair is constantly bending, twisting, & rubbing against other materials so of course the hair will become dry & maybe even a little more course near the ends as time progresses.

Using a deep conditioner product will not be done frequently but it is vital for balancing much needed moisture into your hair extensions when needed. You will usually notice that during the hotter & drier times of year, more deep conditioning is required to quench drier hair!

A good guide for knowing how often to deep condition your hair extensions is at least every two weeks or once a month. Deep conditioning your extensions will vary sometimes depending on how tight your curl pattern is, your hair care styling habits, & usage of other products on the hair as well. If you deep condition non removable extensions, avoid conditioning your scalp to avoid product buildup.

I will walk you step by step through how to deep condition your hair extensions properly from start to finish!

If you are in need of a quality deep conditioner for your extensions, I highly suggest referring to HowToBlackHair.com for suggested product needs.

Deep Condition Regimen
(Removable & Non Removable Extensions)

Step#1 Follow the detangle regimen according to what is applicable for your type of hair extensions.

If applicable, separate & secure away your real hair from your extensions.

Step #2 Saturate your ends with deep conditioner, apply product to the rest of the hair & follow the instructions as suggested.

(Optional) For an intense deep condition, place the extensions in a plastic grocery bag, tie it around the opening of your blow dryer on low to medium heat for 10 minutes.

Step #3 Allow warm water to wash the deep conditioner out of your hair extensions.

Refrain from manipulating or handling your hair while & after rinsing out the deep conditioner.

Final rinse with the coolest water you can stand for smooth shiny hair.

Step #4 (Non Removable Extensions)
Gently scrunch towel dry extensions & allow to air dry with an absorbent towel around your neck.

(Removable Extensions) Hang dry your extensions on pant hangers or dry on top of an absorbent towel.

5 CONDITIONER WASH

The key to keeping hair extensions healthy is to conditioner wash your hair! Keeping your investment moisturized prevents it from becoming chronically dry since the key to great looking hair has always been an incorporation of co-washing. Co-washing your hair means to wash your extensions with conditioner alone. When you are not in need to cleanse your hair, use a moisturizing conditioner instead to freshen up your extensions as well as make them softer & moisturized once again.

The frequency of your co-wash should be at least twice a week or every other day. If you are co-washing non removable extensions, avoid conditioning your scalp to avoid product buildup. To keep your extensions looking fresh & frizz-free throughout the day, you should not rake your fingers through your hair as it is drying! Also as tempting as it may be, refrain from handling curly to coily hair while drying & more importantly when dry, to preserve neat looking extensions.

I will walk you step by step through how to co-wash your hair extensions properly from start to finish!

If you are in need of a quality conditioner for your extensions, I highly suggest referring to HowToBlackHair.com for suggested product needs.

Co-Wash Regimen
(Removable & Non Removable Extensions)

Step #1 On detangled hair, generously saturate your hair with conditioner & then detangle with a seamless wide tooth/detangling comb.

If applicable, separate & secure away your real hair from your extensions.

Step #2 Allow warm water to wash the conditioner out of your hair extensions.

Refrain from manipulating or handling your hair while & after rinsing out the conditioner.

Final rinse with the coolest water you can stand for smooth shiny hair.

Step #3 (Non Removable Extensions)
Gently scrunch towel dry extensions & allow to air dry with an absorbent towel around your neck.

(Removable Extensions) Hang dry your extensions on pant hangers or dry on top of an absorbent towel.

(Optional) Blow dry diffuse your extensions or high ponytail your extensions & then dry with a hooded dryer.

6 MOISTURIZE
(LEAVE IN CONDITIONER)

The amount of leave in moisturizer product you will need to use will vary depending on the quality of health & curl pattern of your extensions. Straight to wavy hair extensions usually requires a small amount of moisturizer while curly to coily hair extensions typically require a little more moisturizer to prevent the hair from dryness.

The frequency of your moisturizing needs should be at least twice a week or every other day. To keep your extensions looking fresh & frizz-free throughout the day, you should not rake your fingers through your hair as it is drying! Also as tempting as it may be, refrain from handling curly to coily hair while drying & when it is dry, to preserve neat looking extensions.

I will walk you step by step through how to moisturize your hair extensions properly from start to finish!

If you are in need of a quality moisturizer for your extensions, I highly suggest referring to HowToBlackHair.com for suggested product needs.

Moisturizing Regimen
(Removable & Non Removable Extensions)

Step#1 On a detangled section of hair, vigorously rub a small amount of moisturizer into your hands & smooth it onto your extensions.

Primarily focus on the extension ends since this is in most need of moisture!

Step #4 (For Non Removable Extensions)
Apply Step #1 in manageable sections to prevent an overlapping of product.

If applicable, separate & secure away your real hair from your extensions.

7 HAIRSTYLING TOOLS

It is completely optional to use hairstyling tools for your hairstyling needs but make sure that your tools are of quality to preserve the integrity of your hair! Depending on your preferences, the look of your hair is always completely up to your imaginations & with high quality hair extensions; you can run wild & do whatever you want to do!

The easiest & best way to wear your hair in a desired hairstyle is to wear your extensions in its natural state. For instance, if you like curly hair, purchase curly hair instead of curling straight to wavy hair for your desired look. The same goes for straight hair, it makes more sense to buy straight hair extensions instead of constantly applying heat to make wavy/curly/coily extensions straight.

I will walk you step by step through a variety of hairstyling options you can do with your hair extensions & I will also help you to distinguish between safe & harsh hair styling tools!

Hairstyling Options
(Removable & Non Removable Extensions)

DEEP WAVES

(Heat) Take chunky sections of detangled hair & press your waver tool near the base of the section near your scalp. Hold for 5-10 seconds & then press your waver again down the section you are working on, making sure that you follow the last wave indent for consistent waves.

(No Heat) Take chunky sections of detangled hair & secure wave rollers onto your sections. You can also achieve waves by braiding chunky braids on damp hair & unravel them when dry.

BEACH WAVES

On small detangled sections, position your flat iron/straightener near the roots of your section with the side of the straighter pointing directly up toward the ceiling while still keeping the plates closed. At this point, your hair is forced upward toward the ceiling too. Slowly & firmly slide your straightener down to the very ends for wide curls. Rake your fingers through all of your curls for beach hair!

SPIRAL CURLS

Use a curling wand for easy uniform spiral curls & wear a protective glove on your less dominant hand. With your dominant hand holding the wand, you have better control in preventing burn accidents. Wrap small to medium sized detangled sections of hair around the wand, hold for 5-10 seconds & then release. Separate curls for bigger hair!

SAFE HAIR STYLING TOOLS	HARSH HAIR STYLING TOOLS
Bobby Pins with Balled Ends	Bobby Pins with no Balled Ends
Silk Accessories	Cotton Accessories
Ouchless/Seamless Hair Bands	Metal/Plastic Binding Hair Bands
Paddle Brush	Metal Wig Brush
Heat Styling up to 350°	Heat Styling over °350
Blow Drying on Low to Medium Heat	Blow Drying on High Heat

8 HAIR CARE REGIMEN (REMOVABLE EXTENSIONS)

The easiest part about caring for your extensions is when they are removable because this gives you the greatest flexibility when it comes to taking care of your real hair & your hair extensions!

The suggested regimen is only applicable when caring for your removable extensions since you are able to care for your hair extensions separately from your real hair.

By using the suggested hair products mentioned in this guide when following the regimen, you will be able to keep your extensions in a healthy condition!

If you are in search of products or information for your real hair, check out HowToBlackHair.com for more information & products to help you keep your hair clean, moisturized & healthy!

Next I will walk you step by step through an easy to follow hair care regimen for removable extensions to keep your extensions looking healthy & beautiful!

Hair Care Regimen (Removable Extensions)
Day 1 Shampoo (Mandatory) Deep Condition (Mandatory) Moisturize (Mandatory)
Day 2
Day 3 Moisturize (If Needed)
Day 4
Day 5 Conditioner Wash (Co-Wash) (Mandatory) Moisturize (Mandatory)
Day 6
Day 7 Moisturize (If Needed)
Week 2 Day 1 Shampoo (Mandatory) Moisturize (Mandatory)

9 HAIR CARE REGIMEN
(NON REMOVABLE EXTENSIONS)

You have already been equipped with a hair care routine for your extensions if they are removable but what about caring for your hair & non removable extensions?

What about if you are wearing a Sew In, Lace Closure, ¾ Wig, Micro Links & even Fusions for example?

The same techniques can be applied to your real hair as well so no more worries about dry breaking damaged hair after removing your extensions!

Since your hair will be covered with extensions for some time, it's urgently important that you take the necessary steps to treat your hair as suggested by the following regimen.

This greatly prevents your hair from breakage, dryness & brittleness while wearing your install!

By using the suggested hair care products mentioned in this guide, you are able to use those same products that are formulated for virgin hair extensions, for your real hair as well!

Next I will walk you step by step through an easy to follow hair care regimen for non removable extensions to keep both your extensions & your real hair healthy & beautiful!

Hair Care Regimen (Non Removable Extensions)
Day 1 Shampoo (Mandatory) Deep Condition (Mandatory) Moisturize (Mandatory) Shampoo, deep condition, & moisturize your real hair first & then perform the same steps on your extensions separately before installing them into your hair.
Day 2
Day 3 Moisturize (Real Hair + Extensions If Needed)
Day 4
Day 5 Conditioner Wash (Co-Wash) Extensions(Mandatory) Real Hair (If Needed) Moisturize Extensions(Mandatory) (Real Hair If Needed)
Day 6
Day 7 Moisturize (Real Hair + Extensions If Needed)
Week 2 Day 1 Shampoo Extensions(Mandatory) Real Hair (If Needed) Moisturize Extensions(Mandatory) Real Hair (If Needed)

10 COLORED HAIR
CARE MAINTENANCE

Caring for colored hair needs to have more incorporation of moisture than that of extensions that are in its natural state of color!

Colored extensions aren't any different than your real hair in a colored state but it is always better to allow your extensions to take to color rather than your real hair.

This offers so much versatility because you can always wear different extensions of different colors as frequent as you want without having to change the color of your real hair!

Colored hair requires more maintenance to keep it healthy & full of body & movement so the same techniques & products will apply to the regimen given on the following page.

By using the suggested hair care products mentioned throughout this guide, you are able to use those same products formulated for virgin hair extensions, for your real hair as well!

Refer to HowToBlackHair.com for formulated hair care products for you real hair if you choose to use different products for your own hair instead.

I will walk you step by step through an easy to follow hair care regimen for maintaining colored hair while keeping both your extensions & your real hair healthy & beautiful!

Colored Hair Care Maintenance
Day 1 Shampoo (Mandatory) Deep Condition (Mandatory) Moisturize (Mandatory) Shampoo, deep condition, & moisturize your real hair first (if applicable) & then perform the same steps on your extensions separately before installing them into your hair.
Day 2
Day 3 Moisturize Extensions(Mandatory) Real Hair (If Needed)
Day 4
Day 5 Conditioner Wash (Co-Wash) Extensions(Mandatory) Real Hair (If Needed) Moisturize Extensions(Mandatory) (Real Hair If Needed)
Day 6
Day 7 Moisturize Extensions(Mandatory) Real Hair (If Needed)
Week 2 Day 1 Shampoo (Mandatory) Deep Condition (Mandatory) Moisturize (Mandatory)

11 HEAT DAMAGED HAIR CARE MAINTENANCE

Caring for heat damaged hair needs to have more incorporation of moisture than that of healthy hair extensions because it's natural ability to retain moisture need to be restored!

In most cases, heat damaged hair is irreversible because the amount of heat placed on the extensions has altered its abilities to retain its natural shape. This is extremely noticeable on hair that is not naturally straight because you will notice straight strands of hair that are resistant to returning to its original shape of a curl/coil/wave!

There is hope in nursing this hair back to health with the chance of weekly mandatory deep conditions. If this does not help restore your hair, you have to call it a loss & take better care of your next set of extensions to avoid this problem!

By using the suggested hair care products from HowToBlackHair.com, you should be able to use those same products that are formulated for virgin hair extensions, for your real hair as well!

Next I will walk you step by step through an easy to follow hair care regimen for maintaining heat damaged hair while keeping both your extensions & your real hair healthy & beautiful!

Heat Damaged Hair Care Maintenance

Day 1 Shampoo (Mandatory)
Deep Condition (Mandatory)
Moisturize (Mandatory)

Shampoo, deep condition, & moisturize your real hair first
(if applicable) & then perform the same steps on your
extensions separately before installing them into your hair.

Day 2

Day 3 Moisturize
Extensions(Mandatory) Real Hair (If Needed)

Day 4

Day 5 Conditioner Wash (Co-Wash)
Extensions(Mandatory) Real Hair (If Needed)

Moisturize
Extensions(Mandatory) (Real Hair If Needed)

Day 6

Day 7 Moisturize
Extensions(Mandatory) Real Hair (If Needed)

Week 2 Day 1
Shampoo (Mandatory)
Deep Condition (Mandatory)
Moisturize (Mandatory)

AFTERWORDS

The Virgin Extensions Hair Care Manual was made to help you take care & maintain healthy hair extensions! You may have chosen to read this guide because you support my work, you were looking for hair care regimens for extensions, or you were looking for this information to help out a loved one.

I personally understand how frustrating it can be taking care of virgin hair extensions but as you may have realized, incorporating a regimen will make maintaining your hair a second nature process! When you are not knowledged about what keeps your extensions healthy & which products are best for your investment, you will often struggle with extensions that have a hard time lasting as long as you hoped for! That is why throughout this guide, I highly suggested hair care products referred from HowToBlackHair.com

This manual was filled up with hair knowledge, styling tips, & amazing hair care regimens that will serve as your go to resource when caring for your extensions as well as your real hair throughout the duration of your hairstyle & beyond! Make sure to come back & review/follow the regimens in this book as often as possible to get the most out of your virgin hair extensions!

Thanks for reading this guide; it was a pleasure of mine to write this for your knowledge & enjoyment."

Sincerely, Breanna

ADDITIONAL RESOURCES

The Official Website: www.Howtoblackhair.com
The Online Store: www.HowtoblackhairStore.com
Free Subscription Email: http://eepurl.com/FZs5b

For Additional Hair Questions
YourHairQuestions@Gmail.com

Black Hair Styling Tutorials

BlackWomenHair YouTube Channel
www.Youtube.com/BlackWomenHair

HowToBlackHair YouTube Channel
www.Youtube.com/HowToBlackHair

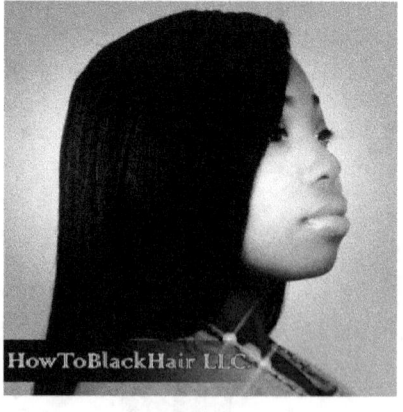

The Natural Hair Bible
The 10 Commandments of Black Hair Care
www.HowToBlackHair.com

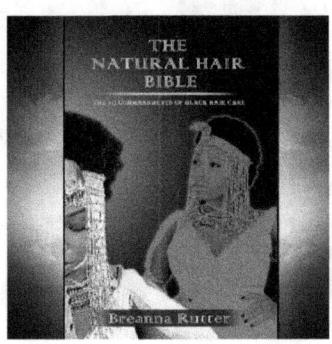

The Black Hair Manual
A Pocket Guide for Choosing Your Best Hair Products
www.HowToBlackHair.com

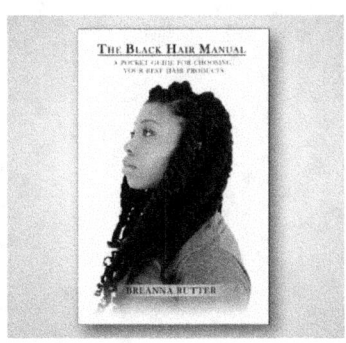

Black Hair Styling DVDs (Over 20+ Hairstyles)
www.HowToBlackHair.com

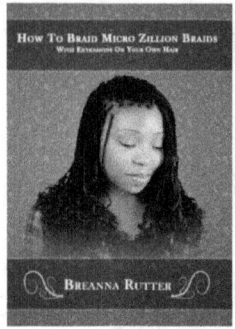 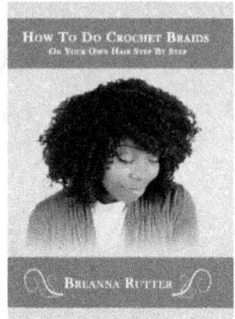

DEFINITION GUIDE

Build Up: *hair care products, sweat, dirt, oils, and/or skin that has gathered on your hair and scalp*

Colored Hair: *hair that has been colored*

Co Wash: *to only wash your hair with conditioner alone for moisture*

Curl Pattern: *the look of your curls based on the LOIS or Andre Walker Hair Typing System*

Damage: *hair that is opposite of a desirably healthy condition*

Detangle: *to free the hair of knots and tangles*

Elongate: *gravity's natural pull on your hair*

Extensions: *hair that is attached to your head for adornment*

Finger Detangle: *using your fingers to gently rake through tangles*

Frizz: *hair with raised cuticle scales and does not look smooth*

Groom: *fashioning your hair in a neat smooth appearance*

Lather: *to produce a frothy airy mass from your hair products*

Matted: *hair that is beyond tangled and nearly impossible to detangle*

Non Removable Extensions: *extensions you choose to leave in for an extended period for the sake of a hairstyle ex; Sew In*

Regimen: *the implementation of hair products and manipulation techniques used for maintaining healthy hair*

Removable Extensions: *extensions you choose to wear temporarily and can be removed and installed again instantaneously ex; Clip Ins*

Retain Moisture: *the ability to keep moisturized hair even after it has dried*

Virgin Hair: *hair extensions that are free of any chemical processing*

Seamless Wide Tooth Comb: *a comb with no seams to be felt within the binding of teeth of the comb that will aggravate your hair and cause breakage*

Split Ends: *the thinning appearance at the end of a strand of hair*

Tangle: *hair that is not free of tangles and knots*

Trim: *to modestly cut off hair usually no more than a 1/8 inch*

INDEX

THE VIRGIN EXTENSIONS HAIR CARE MANUAL

HOW TO BLACK HAIR LLC.

WRITTEN BY BREANNA RUTTER
BOOK DESIGNED BY BREANNA RUTTER
COVER DESIGNED BY JARED RUTTER

ALL RIGHTS RESERVED.

VISIT WWW.HOWTOBLACKHAIR.COM

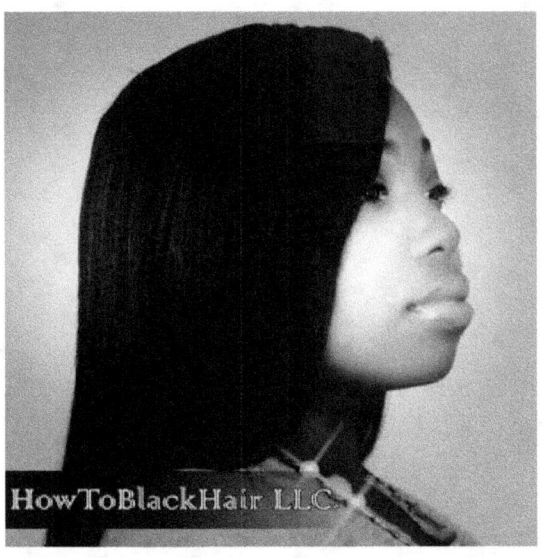